Bruce Wembulua Shinga

Role of IT in the management of Hospitals

GRIN Publishing

GRIN - Your knowledge has value

Since its foundation in 1998, GRIN has specialized in publishing academic texts by students, college teachers and other academics as e-book and printed book. The website www.grin.com is an ideal platform for presenting term papers, final papers, scientific essays, dissertations and specialist books.

Visit us on the internet:

http://www.grin.com/

http://www.facebook.com/grincom

http://www.twitter.com/grin_com

The role of Information Technology (IT) in the management of hospitals: Contribution to the reduction of economic costs.

Dr WEMBULUA SHINGA BRUCE

Student of online Master of Science in Health Management

UNIVERSITÀ TELEMATICA INTERNAZIONALE UNINETTUNO.

This piece of work describes succinctly the role of Information Technology in hospitals and explain by the way how it contributes to the reduction of economic costs in the health sector

Academic year 2016 -2017

INTRODUCTION

The health industry is growing at a feverish pace (Ciampa and Revels 2013: xi). It is estimated that up to 30% of the total health budget may be spent one way or another on handling information, collecting it, looking for it, and storing it (HIQA 2013: 3). In the coming decades, the healthcare system will be undergoing the biggest transformation of any industry in the history (Westbrook 2007). Health being information-intensive, safe and reliable healthcare will depend more and more on access to, and the use of, information that is accurate, valid, reliable, timely, relevant, legible, complete and retrievable. From the care delivery point of view, there will be significant increase in the demand for high quality care. The aging population with more complicated medical problems coupled with the increasing medical knowledge, will demand greater services and effort from limited medical resources (HIQA 2013, Westbrook 2007). Furthermore, the increasing utilization of multidisciplinary care creates the need for interoperability between various healthcare entities. The need for rapid automation of the medical care with new technologies addressing the medical data management is therefore obvious.

Although our current health system in general is inconsistently and significantly underutilizing the Web and IT (Kabene 2010), it is asserted that technology is one of the most pervasive and ubiquitous tools in healthcare today, transforming not only healthcare but also the professions within it (Conrick 2006) by alleviating in certain ways, both financial and management burdens. Information technology (IT) is therefore perceived to possess the potential to improve the quality, safety, and efficiency of health care. Lines below, try to describe how this comes to happen.

CHAPTER 1 : HEALTHCARE IN THE ERA OF ADVANCED IT: OVERVIEW AND EVOLUTION

Purchasing and providing health is an information intensive activity. Having ready access to timely, complete, accurate, legible, and relevant information is critical to health care organizations, providers, and the patients they serve (Wager, Wickham and Glaser 2013), as this sector of our society strives to provide quality care and ensure adequate access. Health informatics referring to the application of information technology in health sector can be defined as a combination of computer science, information science and health science designed to assist in the management and processing of data, information and knowledge to support healthcare and healthcare delivery (Conrick 2006: 4). It is therefore intended to address different challenges that healthcare systems face today, like increasing amount of data and information to manage, the strong need for shortening period of hospitalization through best healthcare delivery, the provision of secure and efficient billing process etc. For this to happen, the computer should offer the healthcare system greater flexibility, efficiency and effectiveness by reducing redundant data, duplicate testing and providing information at the point of care (Conrick 2006).

Reports of using computers to support clinical data management activities date back to the late 1950s (Carter 2008). Over the years systems have been designed to support most activities related to health care business practices and clinical process: Administrative and financial systems to facilitate billing, accounting, and administrative tasks, Clinical systems that provide input into the care process, and Infrastructure that supports both administrative and clinical applications (Kedar and Bhattacharya 2011). At the same time as the demand for adequate information has increased, numbers of advances are registered in information technology applicable to health domains. The development of medical instruments using information technology in a vast number of instances, varying from monitor equipment to CT and MRI scanners. Requirements on the registration and processing of medical services and hospital bills have led to extensive Electronic Data Processing facilities, Hospital Information Systems (HIS) and ancillary registration systems. Largely paper-based medical record system, in which information is often incomplete, illegible, or unavailable where and when it is needed, are being shifted to a system in which the patient's clinical information is integrated, complete, stored electronically, and available to the patient and authorized persons anywhere, anytime (Wager, Wickham and Glaser 2013; Armoni 2000). Standardized records formats, nomenclature, and communication protocols led to the vital notion of interoperability through which providers involved in patient care have immediate access to patients records, electronic decision-support tools, the latest relevant research findings on a given topic, and patient-specific reminders and alerts; the advent of the internet has led to the notion of e-health and powered an era of open access to diverse medical knowledge. Moreover, health care executives should be able to devise strategic initiatives that take advantage of access to real-time, relevant administrative and clinical information (Wager, Wickham and Glaser 2013; Kedar and Bhattacharya 2011).

In health care, many clinical practices are not sustained by scientific evidence either because evidence from well conducted, randomized controlled trials is not available or just as its timely dissemination to practitioners is not ensured. Although the ever growing clinical and biomedical research production, studies suggest that process of transferring clinical evidence from research to practice might take an average of 17 years (Ortiz and Clancy 2003). The use of IT in this context has helped overcome cases of delay, loss, and waste in the production and of evidence from research. Aside from word processing, Internet through electronic mail is by far the commonest computer application that has revolutionized our contemporary way of getting information. This improve the quality of care as the translation, implementation, and dissemination of important research findings in clinical practice becomes easy (Ortiz and Clancy 2003, Donald, Lindberg in Balas 2000).

CHAPTER 2: ELECTRONIC HEALTH RECORDS AND INTEROPERABILITY

The ad hoc collection of health data and the "silos" in healthcare have little place in a modern health system. There are now two powerful drivers shaping the face of health and manner in which data are collected: Electronic Health Records and the need to share data seamlessly across geographical settings (Conrick 2006: 20). EHRs were originally envisioned just as patients' medical data stored in electronic form in replacement of paper-based records. Now they are generally viewed as a part of an automated order-entry and patient-tracking system providing real-time access to patient data, as well as a continuous longitudinal record of their care (Kedar and Bhattacharya 2011). The EHRs can only deliver their expected benefits when the information and the EHR are Standardized and "structured" in uniform ways allowing the system both to send standardized data to and to receive standardized data from other providers (Stroupe 2011). This "send and receive" capability is known as "interoperability". This is viewed as the ability of two or more systems or components to exchange information and to use the information that has been exchanged (HIQA 2013:8). Discussion of interoperability focus on development of standards defining the format of the interoperable data, medical terminologies to use and security and privacy safeguard terms (Stroupe 2011, HIQA 2013). ICD-10, HL7, SNOMED CT are commonly known examples of standardized codes and ISO, CEN, HL7 some standards development organizations.

The benefits of using interoperable EHR systems in healthcare are definitely established, both in terms of healthcare quality and cost effectiveness (Carter 2008). In 2000, the Institute of Medicine (IOM) estimated that approximately 100,000 deaths per year occurred from medical errors, of which 7,000 were attributed to Adverse Drug Events (ADEs) (IOM cited in Stroupe 2011: 6). Moreover, patients have long experienced the frustration and time-consuming task of supplying the same information over and over again to numerous providers, and are often subjected to repeat testing for the same reason, even within a few hours or days or weeks. To address such health care issues many developed countries have been moving toward interoperable electronic records. They Reduce medical errors and prevent drug and allergy interactions by the integration of Clinical Decision Support Systems (CDSS) using advanced technologies such as Computerized provider order entry (CPOE) to provide prescription drug interaction warnings. The Electronic Medication Administration Records (eMAR) ensure that the correct patient receives the proper medication. The Automated dispensing machines (ADMs) can be used to distribute medication doses to minimize over dosage (Stroupe 2011, Carter 2008).

EHRs are viewed as a more robust technology that integrates two or more systems to provide data to a patient's clinical record (Stroupe 2011:4). CPOE Systems provide, in addition to decision support functions, an integrated view of orders and results (medications, radiology, and laboratory). The integration of Picture archiving and communication systems (PACS) allows timely access to radiological images from various devices (X-Ray, MRI, Computed tomography scan). As part of advanced EHR environments, these technologies systematically reduce or eliminate duplicate tests and care, and thereby reduce costs (Stroupe 2011, Carter 2008, Kedar and Bhattacharya 2011). Finally, by providing patients with access to their medical records scattered across multiple provider offices and hospitals, an interoperable EHRs system allows patients to really participate in the care process (Stroupe 2011).

CONCLUSIONS

The modern era of clinical information systems is being driven by concerns of quality, patient safety, and cost, in addition to secondary business and operational issues. Hence, today emphasis has shifted toward providing information systems that support providers during the process of care (Carter 2008). This results in the advent of various technologies (CPOE, PCS, etc.). The increased volume of medical knowledge related to the advent of the internet and the huge volumes of data generated every day by different healthcare processes have so long burdened the health sector affecting both the quality of care and management of the whole health system. In hospitals, the creation of departmental systems followed by their shift from just carrying out administrative tasks to more clinically orientated functions have arose the need for interoperability. The interoperable EHRs taking the place of largely paper-based medical record systems, offer a system in which the patient's clinical information is structured, complete, stored electronically, and available to the patient and authorized persons anywhere, anytime. While used in medical research domains, IT enhances the implementation, and dissemination of important research findings in clinical practice supporting indeed evidence based medicine practice to improve medical care.

Advantages drawn from all these innovations in terms of accuracy, time allocated both to management processes (i.e. planning, decision making or evaluation) and healthcare provision, result in global reduction of economic cost within the hospital in particular and the whole health sector in general. The completeness of data stored on electronic basis and their secure accessibility create a safe administrative environment in which admission, discharge, and transfer processes are easier. Billing and accounting system become henceforth more secure with narrower possibility of mistake. IT has surely the potential to improve the quality, safety, and efficiency of health care. However, the better is to come since its diffusion in the health industry is still low.

BIBLIOGRAPHY

1. Armoni, A. (2000). Healthcare Information Systems: Challenges of the New Millennium. London, Idea Group Publishing.
2. Carter, J.H. (2008). Electronic Health Record: A guideline for Clinicians and Administrators. 2d ed. USA, The American college of physicians.
3. Ciampa, M. and Revels M. (2013). *Introduction to Health Information Technology.* 1st ed. Boston, Course Technology, Cengage Learning.
4. Conrick, M. (2006). Health Informatics: Transforming Healthcare with Technology. Thompson, Social science Press.
5. Donald A.B, Lindberg M.D. (2000) 'transferring research through high performance computing'. In Balas E.A, Boren S.A, and Brown G.D. *Information technology strategies from the United States and the European Union: transferring research to practice for health care improvement.* Washington DC, IOS press.
6. Health Information and Quality Authority (HIQA). (2013). *Overview of health interoperability standards.* [Online] available from <https://www.hiqa.ie/../Health care-Interoperability-Standards.pdf> [20-10- 2016].
7. Institute of Medicine (IOM). (2000). *Medical errors: A look at the IOM report* cited in Stroupe, M. (2011). *What is EHR Interoperability and why should I care?* [Online] available from <www.nethealth.com/wp.../11/What-is-EHR-Interoperability.pdf> [20-10- 2016].
8. Kabene, S.M. (2010). Healthcare and the Effect of Technology: Developments, challenges and advancements. New York, IGT Global.
9. Kedar, P. and Bhattacharya, A. (2011).*Role of information technology in healthcare.* [Online] available from <https://books.google.com.ph/books?isbn=1329498631> [20-10- 2016].
10. Mills, E. et al. Generation Y in Healthcare: The need for new socio-technical consideration for future technology design in Healthcare in Westbrook, J.I. et al. *Information Technology in Healthcare 2007.* (2007) IOS Press.

11. Ortiz, E., Clancy, C. (2003). 'Use of Information Technology to Improve the Quality of Health Care in the United States'. *Health services research* 38(2): xi–xxii [Online] available from https://www.ncbi.nlm.nih.gov/pmc/articles/PMC1360897 > [0-10- 2016].
12. Stroupe, M. (2011). *What is EHR Interoperability and why should I care?* [Online] available from <www.nethealth.com/wp.../11/What-is-EHR-Interoperability.pdf > [20-10- 2016].
13. Wager, K., Wickham, L., and Glaser, P. (2013).*Health Care Information Systems: A Practical Approach for Health Care Management*. 3d ed. San Francisco, John Wiley & Sons, Inc.

YOUR KNOWLEDGE HAS VALUE

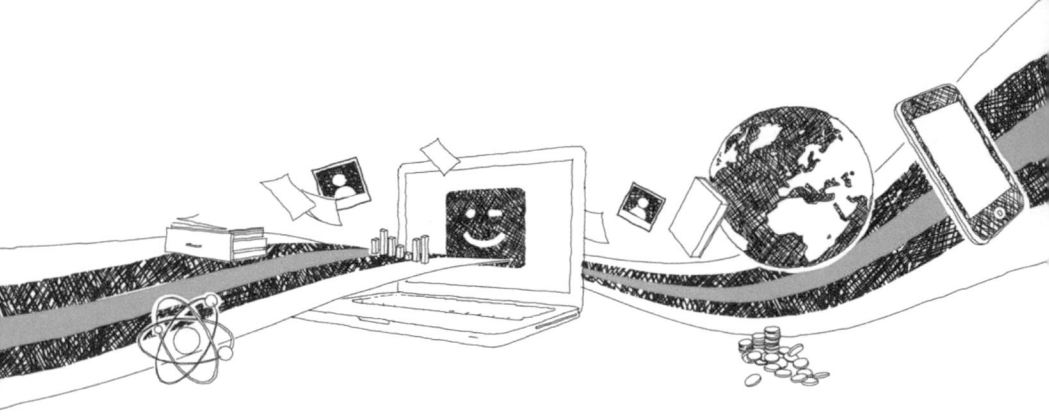

- We will publish your bachelor's and master's thesis, essays and papers

- Your own eBook and book - sold worldwide in all relevant shops

- Earn money with each sale

Upload your text at www.GRIN.com and publish for free

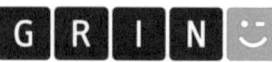